The Enduring Principles of Good Psychiatry

The Enduring Principles of Good Psychiatry

✦

Knowledge, Compassion, and Tenacity

Richard W. Hudgens, M.D.

iUniverse, Inc.
New York Lincoln Shanghai

The Enduring Principles of Good Psychiatry
Knowledge, Compassion, and Tenacity

iUniverse, Inc.

For information address:
iUniverse, Inc.
2021 Pine Lake Road, Suite 100
Lincoln, NE 68512
www.iuniverse.com

ISBN: 0-595-33542-X

Printed in the United States of America

This work is dedicated to Lee Robins and to the memory of Eli Robins, George Winokur and Sam Guze. These four, on the faculty of the Washington University School of Medicine, were among the pioneers in the great work of bringing the world of clinical psychiatry into the world of science, to the benefit of millions.

I write this book with special thanks to Bob Cloninger, Renard Professor of Psychiatry at the Washington University School of Medicine, who provided me with an invaluable opportunity to learn and to teach.

Contents

INTRODUCTION

Psychiatry is the branch of medicine whose practitioners are expected to take responsibility for the care of people who suffer from disorders of thinking, emotions, perception or behavior. This responsibility exists whether the trouble is slight or disabling, whether the cause is known or unknown, and whether or not the affliction occurs in the presence of medical illness or disruptive life circumstances.

Throughout recorded history, long before the word psychiatry was invented, there have been men and women who took on this caring task, conventionally the healers of the community, doctors and priests and those appointed to assist them. Their calling to heal, whether four thousand years ago or now, should be seen as separate from the role of those charged with keeping order in the community—the police and their historical predecessors in the control of disruptive behavior.

It is my belief that despite the many changes in the practice of medicine, the principles followed today by those psychiatrists who take the best care of their patients are timeless, no different now than they were a hundred years ago, and likely no different than those followed by our predecessors in ancient Greece or Mesopotamia. For the essence of doctors' duty has always been to bring three things to their suffering patients: knowledge, compassion, and tenacity. Knowledge to discover what is wrong and what to do about it, compassion to keep the patients' needs ahead of all other considerations, and the tenacity to persist in the work of healing, whatever may block the road. This third quality, tenacity, may be the most important in determining how good a doctor is. Her knowledge will always be incomplete, her compassion will always fall short to some extent, but however relatively ignorant she is, or however relatively short of compassion at any give moment, she should always be able to summon the will to persist in the work of helping her patient.

This book is not about the various psychiatric disorders, their treatment and their cost Readers should look elsewhere for information on those matters. Rather the book is about psychiatrists. I hope the book will help people who are suffering from those disorders of thinking, emotions, perception and behavior—and their families—to know more about what to expect from a psychiatrist so that they will not willingly settle for too little. Medical students, and medical graduates in training to become psychiatrists, may also find it useful.

KNOWLEDGE

The Changing Body of Knowledge and Methods of Inquiry

What new knowledge, relevant to disorders of mood, thinking and behavior, has come into being in the past century; and how has it affected doctors' quest for knowledge about psychiatric illnesses and their treatment of patients?

First, despite what some people today are saying, psychiatric disorders have always in modern times been considered by scientists to be disorders of brain function or structure, or sometimes disorders of other parts of the body expressed through their effects on the brain. For example, neuropathologic discoveries starting in the late 1800's, such as the demonstration that general paresis of the insane was an effect of the organism that causes syphilis, launched such quests as early 20th century searches for the causes of schizophrenia in the microscopic structure of the brain.

In the first half of the 20th century, and a bit beyond, there was a primacy of theories of psychotherapy as the major approach to the understanding the cause and treatment of such illnesses as schizophrenia, bipolar disorder, obsessive compulsive disorder, panic disorder, and major depression. This does not mean that psychiatrists thought brain function was not involved—Freud himself believed there were physiologic causes of psychiatric illnesses—rather it was a reflection of the fact that modern diagnostic methods and pharmacotherapy—treatment with medication—were still in the future. There were no effective means of studying the structure and function of the living brain, nor of treating the illnesses, beyond providing wise counsel, humane conditions for safety and support, and the short-term drug remedies, available for centuries, provided by sedatives and opiates.

The "modern era" of psychiatry may be said to have begun in the third quarter of the 20th century. Psychotherapies of various types and electro-convulsive therapy

1

("shock treatment") were in place by mid-century, and appear here to stay for the foreseeable future. But it was between 1950 and 1975 that all the other current features of assessment and treatment of psychiatric disorders were introduced: an evidence-based method of classifying the types of illness, the beginnings of sophisticated brain-imaging techniques, genetic discoveries, and the development of the drug types known as mood stabilizers, anti-psychotics, and antidepressants.

Despite all the new discoveries about how the brain and the rest of the body look and act physiologically in people with psychiatric illnesses, the principal methods for understanding what is wrong with patients and what to do about it—observing the patient, and taking a history from her and from those who have observed her or treated her previously—are the same as they were a hundred years ago. What is different is the way the psychiatrist organizes the information in her mind and the broader array of treatment options open to her.

What should a patient and the patient's family expect the psychiatrist to know about how to treat her? Having assessed the life situation and diagnosed the condition from which her patient suffers, the psychiatrist should know whether psychotherapy of some type would be helpful, whether or not she herself can provide it, and whether any of a variety of social services are required. She should know whether medication is needed, and if it is, should be able choose from among the four major classes of medication used in psychiatry—antidepressants, anxiolytics (anti-anxiety agents), anti-psychotics, and mood stabilizers—being familiar with the use of several examples of each type of drug. It should be noted here that these categories are not rigidly confined to the actions implied by the labels: antidepressants usually have some anxiolytic action, anti-psychotics often have mood-stabilizing actions, and so forth. The psychiatrist should be aware of this, and aware of the fact that although we think, and organize our understanding of cases, in **syndromes or diagnostic categories**, we treat patients with drugs that relieve **symptoms.**

The psychiatrist should know how the most common "non-psychiatric" conditions, and the means used to treat them, impinge upon psychiatric disorders and their course and treatment. For example, pregnancy, heart disease, hypertension, diabetes, stroke, gastrointestinal complaints and headaches are among the common features of the medical landscape. A psychiatrist who knows essentially nothing of these matters knows too little to practice good general psychiatry.

Are there new psychiatric disorders in these "modern times"? In the broad sense, no. The brain is the brain is the brain, with its standard physiologic and behavioral responses over the millennia to trauma, toxins, starvation, anoxia, physical pressure, external danger, isolation, and loss of care-givers in the broadest sense of the term. But there are new variations on old themes, such as brain infections with brand new agents like the human immunodeficiency virus; and newly refined descriptions of previously recognized phenomena, like post-traumatic stress disorder which has replaced the "shell-shock" syndrome of World War I; and discovery of disorders that may have been there all along unrecognized, like rare genetic aberrations affecting intelligence and behavior.

In general, the disorders that psychiatrists deal with now, whether of mood, cognition, perception or behavior, have been with us from time immemorial. Those not the result of physical insult to the brain such as trauma, infection, or stroke are generally of unknown, or only partly known, causes. When the cause and cure of a psychiatric disorder are discovered and they become preventable, as in the case of general paralysis of the insane, from syphilis, and "myxedema madness" from thyroid hormone deficiency, then responsibility for preventing them becomes the province of other specialists, not psychiatrists.

The Boundaries of Knowledge

As a physician spends time caring for sick people, he becomes more and more impressed with the limits of his knowledge—how very much less he does know than he does not know. This ignorance is both general and specific: how relatively little he knows about people in general and diseases in general, and how incomplete is his knowledge about this particular patient and about the specific disorders that afflict her and the means to help her.

The conscientious physician, daily faced with this reality, will never be satisfied with how much he knows about people and their illnesses, and how to help. He will keep trying to learn more, his efforts limited chiefly by the time and energy available to him. There are two great areas of his ignorance—things that are known by others, but not by him, and things that **nobody** knows. One of his tasks is to try to learn the difference and to remain discontent with the extent of his own knowledge, assuming always that there is much more known than he himself knows.

A lawyer had his first episode of mania, the manic phase of bipolar affective disorder, in his late 20's. On lithium for 30 years, he and his psychiatrist were reasonably satisfied that the illness was adequately controlled, taking into account some elements of mood instability that plague even the most fortunate of those with this bad disease. Then the control began to break down in obvious fashion. There was a succession of job changes, an exceptionally self-destructive love affair, and an irrational demonization of the woman; and then laboratory tests indicated the beginning of impaired kidney function, thought to be in part due to lithium.

During the medication changes made necessary by these developments, he became anxious and confused, and one night he drank a large amount of alcohol and accidentally took double or triple his usual doses of the new medicines. There followed four days in intensive care and a week on a psychiatric division. In the succeeding weeks, as friends and family members weighed in with their observations, it became apparent that for some years preceding these events, things had not been going well with this man. His mood stability, his judgment, and consequently the quality of his life had insidiously worsened, taking him and his psychiatrist by surprise.

With restoration of effective drug therapy by the psychiatrist and frequent common-sense counseling by an experienced therapist matters were put back on track, and life became altogether better than it had been for some time, and kidney function returned to normal.

The incompleteness of the psychiatrist's knowledge, and of knowledge in general, had contributed to different aspects of this crisis. The doctor had not informed himself sufficiently about the whole spectrum of his patient's life, something he could have done. He **had** known that lithium sometimes damages the kidney after many years, but had not predicted it in advance in this man, a prediction that couldn't have been made with current knowledge, though he'd been on the lookout for it and had acted as soon as it was evident.

The Principles of Evaluation and Diagnosis

In the United States a fully trained psychiatrist has completed medical school and at least four years of supervised post-graduate training. These years involve responsibility for taking care of people who have medical and neurological disorders as well as psychiatric illnesses. So patients have a right to expect that the psychiatrist will approach them with a broad view of the possibilities of what may be wrong, and look for troubles that are outside the boundaries conventionally assigned to the field of psychiatry.

In all of medicine, including psychiatry, knowledge has been advanced by the practice of classifying diseases and knowing what happens, right away and over time, when they are not treated—their natural history. A psychiatrist should know how to make a diagnosis of all psychiatric disorders, not necessarily the first time she sees the patient, but certainly very soon. In fact, most psychiatrists can diagnose most mental disorders on the first encounter, or at least narrow the possibilities to such an extent that good treatment can begin. Laboratory studies and psychological tests may be necessary, but in most patients they are not usually important in deciding what the psychiatrist should do first.

The criteria for diagnosing illnesses include a list of symptoms—low mood, insomnia, hearing voices, and so forth—and a chronological account of their appearance. But for a psychiatrist to properly understand what is wrong and what should be done about it he must also know what has been going on in his patient's life, now and in the past—losses, disappointments, hopes, plans, fears—whatever is important to this person he now has the responsibility to help. **For the psychiatrist who is evaluating a patient the narrow act of merely diagnosing an illness is not good enough. An understanding of the patient as a person, in the context of his life past and present, is necessary before the psychiatrist can do the job right. This too can usually be discovered on the first encounter.**

When faced with a patient he has never seen before a psychiatrist must develop a vision as to what level of wellness it is possible for the patient to achieve with respect to relief of symptoms and fulfillment in his life. The patient's vision for himself may have been distorted by the illness, usually in the direction of pessimism, more rarely in the direction of unrealistic euphoria. The psychiatrist can arrive at this vision only as he acquires knowledge of the patient, though information from him or others who have known him. He should then share this vision with the patient himself. It may become a goal that both of them can be guided by.

What about non-psychiatric disorders? Is the psychiatrist supposed to diagnose these, too? Sometimes, yes. And always the symptoms of common non-psychiatric disorders should be inquired about, even if the patient hasn't complained about them spontaneously. The psychiatrist may be the only physician the patient has seen in a long time, and she can assume nothing about the presence or absence of symptoms, nor about the degree of competence and vigilance of the patient's previous doctors. The psychiatrist might herself perform or order the various examinations and tests that will uncover an unsuspected medical or neurological disorder, or may send the patient to another doctor to have this done. Whichever course she takes, it is the psychiatrist's duty to at least consider a non-psychiatric illness when the situation warrants, and to do something about that suspicion.

First Encounter

Doctor and patient approach each other in different moods and with different agendas. The patient is often perplexed and fearful, while the doctor is not. The patient wants his trouble taken away and his mind eased, while the doctor wants information from and about the patient so that she can do that. If the doctor doesn't make it her task at the beginning to discover the patient's specific goals for the visit she cannot serve him well enough, and may go seriously off base.

The patient and his family have the right to expect the same degree of care and systematic vigilance from the psychiatrist whether the first encounter occurs in a quiet office or a busy emergency room. There is no justification for indolence or sloppiness on the part of doctors. Yes, they are all busy, they are human, they have lives of their own, they all get tired, and so on and on. None of these factors counts for much in the face of the patients' needs.

A 35 year old accountant went to a psychiatrist complaining that he was obsessed with the futile quest to get his girlfriend back. He was an anxious man, with a sometime-habit of recreational cocaine. The psychiatrist spent between five and ten minutes listening to him, then told him he had bipolar affective disorder—manic-depressive illness—which was in fact wrong. He wrote five prescriptions: for two antidepressants, one mood stabilizer, one anti-psychotic medication, and one tranquilizer. He told the patient to start taking all five of these at once.

This psychiatrist behaved in ignorant fashion, because he did not take a history, got the wrong diagnosis as it turned out, then prescribed an array of drugs which would have been excessive and risky even if he had been right. He was trying to squeeze so many patients into an hour, to make more money, that he could not do justice to this young man. He is a poster boy for bad psychiatry. Almost as scary, the patient, who was not stupid, obeyed the instructions and soon felt worse, but persisted in following directions for four months. So the case also illustrates the power of a psychiatrist to do harm when his ignorance is coupled with a patient's trust. When a psychiatrist blunders, the results are less likely to be life-threatening than when a surgeon blunders, because of the usually non-fatal nature of psychiatric disorders, even when they are not treated right. But that is small comfort to anyone who is a victim of bad psychiatry.

The psychiatrist's first task is simply to gather information. It is wise for her to talk first to the patient by himself. That starts things off on the right foot, because after all it is the patient himself who is at the center of things. It is he on whose behalf the psychiatrist works and to whom she is ultimately answerable, and whose cooperation she must secure if anything is to get done beyond the first encounter. This goes without saying in those cases when the patient comes to a clinic or a psychiatrist's office on his own initiative for help with a complaint of which he is well aware. But it is of great importance also for children and teenagers, who may have been dragged there unwillingly by their parents, or for patients admitted involuntarily to the hospital, themselves seeing no need for treatment of any sort. What will ultimately drive a case beyond the first encounter is the patient's own perception of a need for continued care. It is best to have the primacy of the patient's concerns considered from the beginning. This lays the groundwork for understanding that the psychiatrist works for the patient, and not the other way around.

There was a time when many psychiatrists were rigid about seeing only the patient, never a member of the patient's family, even if the principle of confidentiality was to be observed. Even those psychiatrists learned to depend on information from others when patients were confused or conspicuously deluded. But in the cases of less disturbed people many psychiatrists would assiduously avoid "contaminating the doctor patient relationship" by talking to a spouse, parent, or other relative even once. Fortunately this practice is going out of style for all but those psychiatrists most lacking in common sense. In many cases it is not necessary to see anyone but the patient, but if there is any evidence or suspicion of severe impairment or incompleteness of information, if marital strife is part of the picture, if the patient is a minor, or if he comes to the psychiatrist accompanied by others, then it is a mistake for the psychiatrist not to avail himself of an additional source of information, even if it is only on the first encounter.

A 50 year old salesman came to a psychiatrist's office complaining of nervousness and asking for medicine to help him sleep. He had no other complaint and blandly answered no to all questions designed to uncover major problems or alarming symptoms. The psychiatrist prescribed something for sleep and walked out to the waiting room with the patient. There he saw the man's wife, whom he hadn't known was there and who seemed eager to talk with him. The patient reluctantly agreed to that. She then told the doctor that her husband had been worrying constantly and unable to work for three months, that she had been trying to get him to see someone, and that he had only agreed that very morning when she had heard him moving around at 4 a.m. and found him in the basement, fastening a rope over a beam to hang himself from.

Instead of walking out of the psychiatrist's office with a sleeping pill, and dangerously suicidal, he walked into the hospital where his depressive episode was treated successfully.

What Must Be Found Out, and How?

The first thing the psychiatrist needs to know is why the patient is there at this particular time. Exploring that it in detail, along with the life situations and the symptoms which preceded the decision by the patient to come (or the decision by others to bring him), will provide the most important information about what is wrong and what to do about it.

One tale which gives a specific account of a specific incident is worth many generalizations. "We fight all the time, and my wife says I nag her, and she's been trying to make me see somebody for a long time," tells the psychiatrist a lot less than, "Well, ok. Last night we got into it when I made her hang up the phone. I think she was talking to some guy she works with. She said I'm crazy, but I found a pen that wasn't mine when I searched her car last night after I got home from work." That specific account gave a solid clue about where the inquiry should proceed in this case of a man who turned out to have a paranoid illness with persistent delusions that his wife was unfaithful. It was not simply "a marriage problem."

The psychiatrist will learn most, and fastest, if she encourages the patient to be spontaneous in a specific account of his symptoms and his life situation. If she jumps in prematurely with a checklist of questions, she may deprive herself of the chance to get the very information that is most important, and may waste time as well.

A good psychiatrist will always ask about important symptoms of various disorders of thinking, mood, and behavior, if that information has not already come out during the patient's spontaneous account. Be skeptical of the common sense and knowledge of any psychiatrist if, in the course of hearing about anxiety and depression, for example, he fails to find out about the presence or absence of alcohol and drug use; suicidal thoughts and acts, past or present; memory problems; fears, odd or reasonable; suspicions, odd or reasonable; job, school or family problems; changes in energy, sleep, appetite and enjoyment. And be highly skeptical of the common sense and training of any psychiatrist who simply sits and stares at his patient, wordlessly, expecting I guess for the patient to read his mind. So much information needs to be gained before help can effectively be delivered, that there is no time for guessing games, or for the psychiatrist to adopt the stereotyped and long-outmoded role of aloof observer.

Psychiatrists are physicians, and they need to know everything about their patients' medical history, currently and in the past, and to look for troubles beyond the boundaries of psychiatry. This cannot be done unless the psychiatrist takes a careful history of physical symptoms, keeping in mind, especially, the common "non-psychiatric" illnesses, and always asking herself, "What might be wrong with this patient besides what I **think** is wrong."

A 33 year old sergeant in the Air Force was arrested for peeking in a neighbor's window. He told the doctor who examined him before his court martial that he was roaming about the neighborhood and looking in women's windows because he was nervous, jittery, too restless to stay home, and had lost a lot of weight in the previous three months. The psychiatrist noticed that his skin was warm and his pulse very rapid. Laboratory tests soon showed that he had an extremely overactive thyroid gland, which warranted immediate treatment.

An elderly man gradually lapsed into depression over a period of several months. He was tired, weak, gloomy in his outlook, and wanted to die. About twenty years before he had been depressed in this way and had recovered after a course of electro convulsive therapy. The patient was resistant to seeing a psychiatrist again, not wanting to undergo the same treatment and hopeless about the outcome in any case. Finally his son persuaded him to go. Seeing him seated beside his healthy son, the psychiatrist noticed how deathly pale he was. A blood count that same day showed that he was profoundly anemic. He had been bleeding from a cancer in his colon. Transfusion, followed by surgery for a cancer that proved non-invasive, cured the man's severe depression, without even one antidepressant pill passing his lips, or even one volt of electricity grazing his temples.

So be skeptical also of the common sense and knowledge of any psychiatrist who fails to ask about past and present medical or surgical illnesses, including injuries, and about those physical symptoms which can appear in either psychiatric and medical disorders: pain anywhere, especially the head, chest, and abdomen; changes in weight; trouble breathing; trouble walking; weakness, general or localized; loss of consciousness, brief or prolonged; problems seeing or hearing or talking or swallowing or urinating; changes in bowel function; problems with sexual function. It doesn't take a doctor long to ask about these matters if the patient has not mentioned them, and it's a serious omission for the doctor to ignore them.

Mutual Education: The Beginning of the Partnership

The doctor and the patient have a lot to teach each other. The illness, or the social turmoil, or whatever problem is uncovered and diagnosed, is going to be the patient's burden to carry. He more than anyone must come to understand it and have a strategy for dealing with it. So above all, a conscientious psychiatrist is going to strive to make the patient his colleague, in effect. Be skeptical of the intelligence of any psychiatrist who doesn't behave in a way that promotes this partnership. What the patient and her family know should be shared with the psychiatrist, beginning his education on the case, and what the psychiatrist knows about the patient's illness, and what he has learned about the patient herself, he should share with his patient, including the name and nature of the disorder, or the environmental stress, he is treating and the options available for dealing with it, with firm recommendations about what he thinks will help most.

The manner and extent of the educational process will depend on the age of the patient, the degree of sophistication of her or his relatives, and the patient's intellectual and emotional ability to take it in. It is a process that begins as soon as the patient is seen, but one that may extend over weeks or even years. The educational process is mutual. The doctor and the patient are both learning as they go along, and in a very real sense, each is the other's teacher.

A 19 year old woman was home for the summer from her college 500 miles away. Her grades had dropped during the semester just ended because she could not concentrate or sleep well. She had broken up with her boyfriend at college after several weeks of arguments over trivial matters. She was crying at slight provocation and keeping to herself. She has never been like this before. She knew something was wrong with her. Her physical examination, done by her family doctor, and laboratory results including tests for thyroid disease and for anemia, were normal.

She had major depressive disorder. In the hour or so it took the psychiatrist to make this diagnosis he also explained what this illness was, as best could be known, and why he believe it was depression and not something else, and what it was going to take to control it: pills, and talking about the issues in her life. She understood and was also provided with written information about depression.

Patients like that are easy to help. They know they are not themselves, they want something done about it, and they are usually open to an explanation that rings true, as long as the psychiatrist has proven himself to be a good listener. In the case of other patients, the educational process is far more difficult and prolonged. *When Ken was 16, he became depressed. His parents took him to a psychiatrist who put him on an antidepressant, and he became better. Then when he was 19, a student in a music conservatory, he began to believe that other people were in some way making him think and do things according to their wishes, not his. He could hear them talking about it, even when no one was there. He did not believe that he was ill, nor that he needed medication.*

The psychiatrist's first task, after eliminating other causes of the symptoms, was to educate the young man's parents about schizophrenia and to begin the process of educating the patient himself. This involved some reading, but mostly it involved one-on-one conversations among the patient, his family, and the psychiatrist, and other mental health professional associates working with the psychiatrist.

Gradually over a period of two years the patient, who had at first taken medication grudgingly, began to attribute his improvement to it. He could see that whereas he had dropped out of school because of his eccentric beliefs, he had now returned to school and achieved a degree. In spite of his feeling, impossible for him to explain, that he was part of someone else's cosmic plan, the medication enabled him to concentrate on the tasks at hand. He was happy with his success and came to see the medication as an aid to concentration and shutting out extraneous voices. So he took it willingly now, though still not certain that his delusions and hallucinations were not real.

Now, over 20 years later, better still because of more effective medications, he has a masters degree, teaches music, plays in a band, and works full time. He knows he has schizophrenia, and he knows what it is, in some ways better than the psychiatrist who started him on the road to controlling it, because it is he himself who has the inside view of the illness.

Having a psychiatric illness is a learning process, and it may take years for a patient whose illness is chronic and marked by a departure from reality, to achieve a productive understanding of what is wrong and what to do about it—to become the doctor's colleague in the treatment of his illness. Many never get that far, but it is a goal for the psychiatrist to strive for always.

All during the process of evaluation and treatment, the psychiatrist and his patient are teaching each other. But it is not, of course, the psychiatrist only who does the teaching about technical matters concerning the illness and its treatment. Information about psychiatric disorders is widely available in books, in the media, and on line. Intelligent patients and their families avail themselves of this information, and may come to know more about a subject than the psychiatrist. Be skeptical of any psychiatrist who is threatened or put on the defensive by what his patient wants to tell him about new discoveries and other matters that pertain to his treatment.

When the patient is himself in the medical profession, the psychiatrist needs to pay special attention to what he says about the subject of his illness.

A 30 year old medical student had suffered from depression for several years, finally having to take a leave of absence from school. When the symptoms were in remission he returned to school, but insomnia, present since the illness began, persisted. Various medications and the institution of sleep-hygiene methods failed to produce adequate sleep and often had troublesome side effects.

He had a long history of the use of sleeping pills, and now withdrew himself from all medications against his nervous psychiatrist's advice. Long after the expected period of withdrawal from sleeping pills he was still not sleeping more than two or three hours a night, despite the lack of any other symptom of either mania or depression. He pro-

duced evidence from the medical literature to support his contention that the period of withdrawal from some drugs commonly used for sleep could last many months. Waiting it out was rewarded: after seven months without medication, using only the routine practices of good sleep hygiene, a normal pattern of sleep was restored.

Psychiatrists are well advised to understand that they don't know everything, and should avail themselves of new information gladly and give a hearing to those who want to teach hem, particularly their own patients

The Enduring Principles of Treatment: The Application of Knowledge to the Relief of Suffering

Treatment begins when the psychiatrist and her patient complete the evaluation, and the psychiatrist has begun to know the patient as a person and to know what is wrong with him.

The first thing that should then happen takes place within the psychiatrist's mind before any therapy is recommended and before any pill is prescribed: she begins to make a prediction about the outcome. The accuracy of this prediction depends upon how much the psychiatrist knows about this illness, or this sort of life-problem, and how well she knows the patient—knowledge always somewhat incomplete. In the normal course of a psychiatrist's professional life, she should get better and better at this as she grows in the profession and as a woman. If she makes the effort, and if she and her patients are fortunate, the older she gets the wiser she will get, the more she will learn, and the more caring she will become.

Why is making a prediction important? Because it sets before the psychiatrist a goal, a vision of how good things should become with respect to the quality of this particular patient's life and his freedom from suffering. The patient himself has come to the psychiatrist with his own vision of how things are and how they are going to turn out. His vision is often narrow and gloomy in the extreme, or frightful, or wildly irrational.

It is the psychiatrist's job to bring hope and reason to bear on the situation and help the patient in his journey toward realistic goals of wellness formulated in the course of their conversations together. The hope within the psychiatrist, born of a realistic vision of her patient's eventual freedom from suffering, can show in her face and her confident manner. This communicates hope to her patient, even before she speaks words of realistic reassurance.

The Natural History of Illnesses

One way the psychiatrist makes predictions is by knowing the natural history of the disorders he treats.

By the late 19th century, more rigorous descriptive studies were underway of people suffering from mental illnesses. Emil Kraepelin, for example, followed for years severely ill patients who had what we now call schizophrenia and bipolar affective disorder (manic depressive disorder). Since the middle of the 20th century, such studies have increased in number, begun by researchers in Europe and North America, whose work was then taken up by workers in other parts of the world.

In the 1950's the psychiatric faculty at Washington University in St. Louis and researchers elsewhere began to pull together the results over the previous half century and to conduct studies of their own. Using description of patients' symptoms, follow-up over years, and studies of patients' relatives, they gathered enough information to create criteria for diagnosing just over a dozen psychiatric disorders and roughly predict their course, untreated, over time. Major depression, bipolar disorder (manic depression), schizophrenia, obsessive compulsive disorder, panic disorder, phobias, generalized anxiety disorder, delirium, dementia (loss of cognitive function), antisocial personality disorder (associated with criminality) somatization disorder (with multiple chronic physical complaints in the absence of objective evidence of physical diseases), substance abuse disorders, mental retardation, eating disorders (anorexia nervosa and bulimia)—the symptoms of all these had been noted for hundreds of years. What was new was the organization into categories that could be studied clinically, biologically, and genetically, leading to understandings of cause and more effective treatments.

Such studies also took into account that these diagnostic categories were not necessarily uniform: for example, there was more than one clinical type of schizophrenia, and different causes each of dementia, delirium, and mental retardation.

A look at the latest edition of the Diagnostic and Statistical Manual used by psychiatrists in the United States informs us that the disorders listed above are by no means the only phenomena considered psychiatric illnesses, only the most important and the best studied. There are hundreds now, including illnesses chiefly observed in children and personality disorders, which are chronic maladaptations mostly described by adjectives—histrionic, explosive, passive-aggressive, and so forth.

In addition, information has been gathered to help doctors know which clinical factors in each illness predict a good outcome, and which a poor one. For example, and not surprisingly, alcohol- or drug-dependence complicating any other psychiatric illness, makes for a worse outcome; the absence of delusions (false beliefs) or hallucinations (false perceptions like "voices") predicts a better outcome for any illness than does the presence of those symptoms in the same type of illness; poor social adjustment in the years before an illness begins predicts a more severe course; disorders with slow ("insidious") onset have a worse outlook than disorders of the same degree of severity with sudden onset. And so on for many psychological, medical, and social factors that precede or accompany the illnesses. It is very important for the psychiatrist to be familiar with these general predictors, even though they cannot be expected to hold up as certain for an individual case.

When Linda was 16, she thought she was plump, so she started to diet and exercise. Sometimes, if she had skipped lunch and gorged on fast foods after school, she would vomit to keep from absorbing those unwanted calories, but this only happened a couple of times a week. She was 5' 5" tall and her weight dropped from 145 to 110 in four months, then leveled off. She began to be fretful and irritable and hard to satisfy, picking fights with her parents and friends. Her mother, observing her moodiness and weight loss, became alarmed. Visions of skeletal anorectics danced through her imagination, like ghostly refugees from a concentration camp.

Her mother dragged her to a psychiatrist. Talking with the girl alone, then together with her mother, the psychiatrist discovered: she had been quite well adjusted in all respects before weight loss began; her weight had leveled off for the previous six months, and her mood had not been getting worse in that time; she was satisfied with her current 110 pounds and wasn't afraid of getting fat; menstruation had not been interrupted; she did not drink alcohol, smoke tobacco or marijuana, or take laxatives, diuretics or diet pills; she rarely vomited; she did not skip school or shop-lift. In sum, none of the bad prognostic indicators of eating disorders were present.

*The psychiatrist knew that this was going to turn out just fine, and his optimism showed in his face as he told the girl and her mother so. Ahead was some counseling, maybe medication. But victory was certain. Of course, that didn't mean that she wouldn't suffer an episode of depression or anxiety later in her life, any more than it meant she would not be killed in a car wreck the next week. But **this particular battle** was all but won.*

On the other hand, consider another woman, who came to the same psychiatrist:

She was 40, a licensed clinical social worker. She told the psychiatrist that she had had anorexia nervosa since she was in her teens and had been a regular drinker as well. The drinking had escalated in volume, and for five years she had been undeniably dependent on alcohol, even driving her children from school drunk on occasion. Her drinking was a secret guarded closely by her, and came to the attention of her husband and family physician surprisingly late. When it did, they ganged up on her and pushed her into an alcohol rehabilitation program. This "took." She became devoted to her recovery through that program and Alcoholics Anonymous.

But all was far from well.

Though she was very thin and had never been otherwise, her terror of becoming fat and her intolerance of any feeling of fullness led her to severely restrict the amount she ate, to vomit repeatedly after each meal, and to take laxatives. All this led to malnutrition and a depletion of potassium in her body which threatened her life. She concealed these self-destructive behaviors from her family and her doctor, who pursued a search for rare metabolic diseases to explain the derangement of her blood chemistry, unaware that the patient was causing this herself. Curiously, depression and a wish to die were not prominent in the clinical picture.

With regard to prognosis, this was a case altogether different from the one before it. There were features that predicted a tough course ahead: anorexia nervosa which was not merely of the food-restricting type, but which also included frequent purging; a history dating back a quarter of a century; the ingestion of large amounts of electrolyte-depleting laxatives, even more dangerous than her former ingestion of alcohol; fearfulness of food and fatness to an irrational degree; the belief, so entrenched as to amount to a delusion, that she was overweight; and a life of deception of her family and her physician to which these fears drove her.

When this came fully to light, no exhortation or threats by her family drove the woman to change any of it.

Hearing all this, the psychiatrist knew it might turn out badly. To prevent that he had to get immediate and firm control of this woman's self-destructive behavior, whatever it took to do that, and ultimately persuade his patient to become his colleague in a life-saving endeavor that flew in the face of her fears. Her behavior was driven by a kind of madness, which had to be greatly reduced in intensity before healing could begin. At the very least the long process of treatment leading to healing would require stubborn endurance by all concerned; hospital treatment at the start, medication, a nutritionist, counseling, and incorporation of the attack on her self-destructive behavior into her Alcoholics Anonymous program. The psychiatrist's task was to convince the patient and her family of the gravity of the situation, and at the same time see the hope of recovery, believing in that himself, and holding that always before the eyes of the patient and her family.

The Natural History of People

The outcome of the troubles people face is not only predicted by the illness they may have, but also by resources of their personality, their maturity, age, intelligence, flexibility, history of coping with bad times, and the presence or absence of family and friends to give them support of all kinds. The psychiatrist should acquire the knowledge of these realities early in the process of treatment and be guided by them in making her predictions.

Consider the stories of two different couples who were referred to the same psychiatrist in the same week.

Susan and Jack, in their 50's, had been married to each other for over 20 years. Both were stable, flexible, and employed in jobs with responsibility for supervision of sizable co-workers. The marriage had been marked by harmony and good health and an absence of marital separation or substance abuse.

On a business trip overseas Jack had an affair with a woman who lived in that country. This was his first misbehavior of that sort. It began at a cocktail party and ended on his initiative two days later, while he was still there. A week after he returned he received an e-mail from the woman on his home computer, which his wife read. She was hurt, furious, threw things and threatened divorce.

They came to a psychiatrist together, with the aim of helping their marriage.

Taking into account all the strength and motivation of them both, and the absence of negative predictors like past instability and substance abuse, the psychiatrist knew that this one should turn out well; that both partners could come out of the crisis wiser and stronger; and that the anger, grief and guilt engendered by this would run their course, if nobody behaved in a way that would prolong them. The psychiatrist's job was to have a vision of harmony restored, to impart that vision to the couple, who were perhaps too distraught to perceive it, and to promote healing, mobilizing the couple's basic respect and compassion for each other.

By contrast, consider Ralph and Carolyn, also in their 50's.

They had been married for six years, and both had been married twice before. Neither had a problem with substance abuse. Ralph worked hard, traveled, and even before their marriage had usually had one or another girlfriend in another city. Carolyn had grown children by an earlier marriage and had not worked since she became pregnant in high school, interrupting her education. She was afraid to be alone, which led to frequent arguments between her and Ralph.

The crisis that led them to a psychiatrist was her accidental discovery of one of his infidelities, the first she had ever known of. Like the other couple they were motivated to save their marriage.

The psychiatrist knew that this was a tougher matter than the first case. There was a husband who habitually fooled around, whatever sterling qualities he may have possessed, and a wife who had not, in a half century of living, yet achieved self-sufficiency and the security that can come with it. The prospects for harmony in this marriage were not bright, even if the flagrancy of his infidelity were to remain a secret. But it was the psychiatrist's job to have a vision of hope and to hold it before the discouraged couple.

"First, do no harm." The doctor knew that if she opened this all up to them together in detail she might sabotage the whole business. Aside from the marriage conflict itself, Ralph and Carolyn had entirely different issues and must work on them as individuals, perhaps with different therapists, for things to be set right between them.

Prediction of probable outcome, based on knowledge of the history of people and their afflictions, governs the psychiatrist's attitude to a case, the degree of hope within her, her ability to sell that vision to her patients, and her choice of the means of solving the problem.

CHOICE OF TREATMENTS

Psychotherapy

Psychotherapy is a term with a long history that has been used to describe so many different techniques of such varying degrees of intensity that many now see it as a generic term meaning almost any treatment that consists of talking between therapist and patient, or between therapist and patients, plural, in a group setting.

It is commonly said that most "talk therapy" is not done by physicians specializing in psychiatry, but by others in the mental health professions who devote full time to it—clinical psychologists, social workers, and counselors—and that most psychiatrists don't do much psychotherapy at all. The first part of that statement is certainly true, in terms of hours spent per patient. But it is not true, or certainly shouldn't be, that psychiatrists don't do psychotherapy.

The verbal interaction that takes place between psychiatrist and patient is the main thing going on, and it underlies everything else that is happening—prescription of medication, psychological testing, physical examination, and so forth. These conversations between physician and patient, however long they last and however infrequently they occur, should be therapeutic in their purpose, centered on the patient's life, symptoms and goals. They are the pathway to mutual education between the doctor and her patient and the means by which the doctor finds out what to recommend and the patient moves toward fuller understanding of himself and the problems he faces, whatever the nature of his symptoms of mood, thinking, perception and behavior. If the psychiatrist does not use the time with her patent in this therapeutic way, however brief the contact, she is not doing her job as well as she should. Similarly, she will not be doing her job as well as she should if she doesn't recognize the necessity, when it arises, of referring some of her patients for more intensive or different psychotherapy which she herself hasn't the time or expertise to provide.

As more conventionally understood, however, psychotherapy consists of regularly scheduled sessions, usually not more than a month apart, and sometimes as frequent as several times a week. What takes place in those sessions varies according to the therapist and the type of therapy employed, and it ranges from the free association of psychoanalytic treatment wherein the patient says everything that comes to his mind thus opening up a world of inner complexities for interpretation, to the relatively structured sessions of cognitive-behavior therapy, which focus on specific items of emotion and behavior to be challenged and changed. Many therapists, whether or not they are physicians, take a flexible approach and devote the sessions to pragmatic consideration of current problems and goals, promoting reflection on past and present events and on the patients' interaction with important people in their lives, a central feature of interpersonal psychotherapy. The aim of psychotherapy is not confined to the elimination of symptoms like depressed mood, anxiety and obsessions, but includes the achievement of the patient's fullest potential.

Does psychotherapy work? And can it hurt? Yes to both questions.

Patients will of course credit psychotherapy for their improvement if they get well or better while the therapy is going on. But apart from that, which by itself proves nothing, controlled research studies of interpersonal therapy and cognitive-behavior therapy have demonstrated their effectiveness in many people with symptoms of anxiety, depression, eating disorders, obsessions and compulsions, with and without the concurrent use of medications.

Interpersonal psychotherapy, a term with a long history, has come to mean a series of meetings in which therapist and patient explore the latter's life—past, present and future—with a focus on his interaction with others and the thoughts and emotions involved in those relationships. From insights gained in this process should come more fulfilling relationships and reduction of emotional distress. Interpersonal therapy can be limited to a specific number of meetings agreed to at the beginning, or be open-ended.

Much interpersonal psychotherapy takes place in the absence of psychiatric illness, though some degree of emotional distress and dissatisfaction with himself drives the person to seek help. The process in its most extensive form is a project of several years' duration, with meetings between therapist and patient at least once a week. It can become the main thing in the patient's life, bonding him to the therapist as confidant, guide, and even judge, whether or not the therapist takes a directive approach in the interaction with his patient. When the patient's life goes well as therapy proceeds, he credits the therapy for his success. It may certainly be true, but there is no way to rerun the process as a controlled experiment.

Very often, though, therapy begins during an episode of illness and continues after the illness has improved or ended:

Marian was 17, a senior in high school, when she first became seriously depressed. The routine frustrations of life suddenly assumed massive significance for her. She cried at the drop of a hat, she couldn't concentrate on studying, she drank herself to sleep every night. The medication part of helping her was the easiest part, but only the beginning. After her symptoms had abated and she was back on track in school she decided to face issues that had been at the back of her mind for some time, and which (who knows?) might have been factors in the onset of her depression: the use of alcohol to help her sleep, the secret power struggle between her and her older brother to be the one anointed to lead the family business, the growing recognition of her own homosexuality and its social consequences. She could speak of none of this to her family, and friends were of dubious help or trustworthiness.

Over the next eight years she was in therapy with a psychiatric nurse who also had training in counseling. They met once a week at first, later about once a month but with a return to the once-a-week schedule during times of change and stress. She could open up about anything without fear of shame or retribution. The therapist became for Marian a touchstone of common sense and reality. "You make me think" she told her. The life-decisions over the eight years of therapy and her growth into a career and satisfying relationships were very much Marian's own doing, not reflecting any goals the therapist—or her family—might have set for her. Would her successes have occurred without therapy? Nobody thinks so, least of all Marian.

Cognitive-behavior therapy takes a two-pronged approach to anxiety and depression. In a systematic and often time-limited series of sessions the patient explores his negative memories and expectations, and the fears, that underlie his distressing symptoms. These are countered with concentration on their positive counterparts—pleasant memories, optimistic expectations. Then the patient acts on the positive expectations, reversing the process of behavioral timidity and withdrawal into anxiety and gloom. Most of the work of cognitive-behavior therapy is homework: the patient confronts himself and builds his lists of positive and negative thoughts, his own cognitions. And it is the patient who puts his positive expectations into action away from the therapy sessions. No one can do it for him.

Following an automobile accident Sunny, a 47 year old woman, developed a fear of driving and would not do so for a period of several months despite the pleas and encouragement of her family, and despite the considerable inconvenience caused by her phobia. There was no benefit to her from her refusal, such as money, sympathy, or getting out of unpleasant tasks. It was simply the stark terror of driving itself. She was highly motivated to get over it as soon as possible.

She and her therapist, a psychologist, worked out a graded series of behaviors, from the least fearful (sitting at the wheel of a stationary car) to the most fearful (merging at the speed limit onto an interstate highway during rush hour). She continued at each level until she could accomplish that task with enough ease that she was willing to go to the next level. By seven weeks she had achieved her goal of driving anywhere, though not without some residual anxiety. The therapist had seen her once a week during that time, helping her counteract her predictions of disaster with reasonable expectations of what was likely once she was free of the phobia, focusing the discussion on the prescribed behavior and the benefits of freedom from fear, always encouraging and optimistic of outcome, emphasizing the patient's strengths, and never pushing her impatiently. After the achievement of the goal, therapy sessions ended, but Sunny has continued to work on decreasing her anxiety by never avoiding driving, even under challenging conditions. Her treatment, graded exposure to feared situations, had desensitized her to those situations and the fear they inspired.

It is standard practice for the psychiatrist to do at least supportive psychotherapy with patients for whom they are also prescribing medication, including even disorders with psychotic symptoms—delusions and hallucinations. This has been associated with better compliance with treatment and accordingly, better results.

Dennis is 44 and has had a particularly disabling case of schizophrenia since he was 19. In the early years of his illness he was uncooperative with treatment, not understanding why he needed medication and not liking his first psychiatrist, who was too busy to spend time talking with him. His new psychiatrist, whom he first saw when he was 30, was more patient with him, taking time to find out Dennis's objections to medication and adjusting the drugs accordingly. In addition, he spent some time at each visit in relaxed conversation about subjects of interest to Dennis. The result:

Dennis became a partner in his own treatment, and while he had been in the hospital five times in the first 12 years of his illness, he has had only one hospital admission in the last 15 years.

How can psychotherapy hurt? In at least two ways. First, when it is used as the only treatment when the patient also needs medication, either because the therapist does not understand the illness he is dealing with, or settles for insufficient symptom relief in the belief that psychological discomfort is essential to the progress of psychotherapy.

A famous lawsuit several years ago, alleging negligence, was resolved in favor of the plaintiff in the case of a physician who was hospitalized for a long period of time and treated only with psychotherapy without success, later recovering promptly on antidepressant medication from a different psychiatrist. This was a wake-up call for any psychiatrist or therapist who had missed, or discounted, the discoveries of the previous half century.

And second, the process of psychotherapy can be harmful if its done wrong. Both therapist and patient should keep the goals of therapy in mind, and it is the therapist's job to remind herself and her patient of this if things get off track. A good working relationship is essential to the success of therapy, and patients often develop strong feelings for and about the therapist. These emotions stem from the patients' hopes and needs and their perceptions of the therapist, whether distorted or not, and often replicate feelings about other important people in their past or current lives. It can be useful for the therapist and patient to discuss this "transference" phenomenon if has resulted in feelings and beliefs that are getting in the way of the goals of therapy. Obviously, negative feelings can block the trust and confidence that are essential to success in therapy. Positive feelings, like those for a dear parent or lover, can be just as problematic if the patient comes to view therapy as an end in itself rather than a means to an end. In such a case the therapist must help her patient keep focused on goals, which invariably should involve "getting a life" beyond the process of psychotherapy itself.

I don't believe it is usually necessary to invoke the psychoanalytic concept of transference to explain patients' feelings about their therapists. A patient can perceive for himself when a therapist is courteous or rude, warm or cold in manner, attentive or bored. If both the therapist and the patient's father, for example, was one of the above, then that just makes two of them. No fancy theory is required to explain the patient's positive or negative reactions.

Glenda, in her early 50's, suffered greatly from grief after her husband died. The first counselor to whom she was referred was inappropriately aloof, at least for Glenda. He allowed long and uncomfortable silences to occur, holding out for more spontaneity and initiative than his patient was capable of. Her grief was in no way lessened.

She switched to a therapist recommended as warm by a friend. This man, whom she saw twice a week for over two years, became the center of her life. She lived for their sessions. During her long and childless marriage she had never been very independent: her life had revolved around her husband, from whom she was rarely away. Now instead of developing independent activities and new social connections as a widow, she withdrew. Habitually rising as late as 11:00, she did the minimum necessary during the day.. By late afternoon she began extended hours of TV and wine, resulting in a pleasant buzz that lasted till bedtime. But she never missed an appointment with her therapist, always arriving on time, nicely dressed and made up.

Her therapist negligently let this go on, without even the excuse of inexperience. She was a paying customer. Also he enjoyed the sessions, as she had warmed to his caring manner, and now opened up her heart endlessly on subjects ranging from her husband, to her childhood, to movies, to politics—everything. Some people, talking chiefly of themselves and their thoughts about this and that, never run out of things to say. He basked in her adulation and never explored with her, much less challenged, her increasing isolation and descent into alcohol dependence, a new prison, replacing her grief, but just as confining.

Medication

The use of drugs to treat psychiatric symptoms is as old as recorded history. Extracts of some plants and various fermented or distilled liquids were discovered thousands of years ago to have sedative, analgesic, and euphoriant properties. Their use will continue as long as there are people on the earth. Since the 19th century there has been increasing scientific research on this pharmacotherapy of emotional, cognitive and behavioral symptoms, so that doctors may move beyond folklore and reliance on anecdotal information to make decisions about treatment.

The second half of the 20th century saw a great increase in the types and numbers of medications used by psychiatrists. The symptoms targeted for attack have been depressed mood, excessively elevated mood and extravagant behavior, instability of mood or action, anxiety and fearfulness, obsessions and compulsions, delusions (irrational beliefs), hallucinations (perceptions, for example, of sounds and sights in the absence of outside stimuli), aggressive feelings and behavior, low energy and behavioral inertia, poor concentration or attentiveness, memory loss, and confusion. Some drugs are naturally occurring substances, some are synthetically produced. Some drugs intended for one use were discovered unexpectedly to have an additional, very different use. Some drugs were designed and manufactured and useful for the purposes intended.

As noted above, psychiatrists think in terms of diagnoses and syndromes—symptom clusters- or they should. But when they give medication they are treating symptoms, and should have no illusion that they are curing the underlying illness. Antipsychotic medications are prescribed for delusional beliefs whether they occur in someone with schizophrenia or severe depression; the mood stabilizer lithium is prescribed for people with bipolar disorder, but also to enhance the effective of other drugs in the treatment of depression; some of the drugs designed for treatment of epilepsy are effective as first-line mood stabilizers. And so on.

A psychiatrist, or anyone else who treats people for mental disorders is behind the times if he says he "doesn't believe in drugs." They are not always necessary, but they often are. He needs to be familiar with the uses and dangers of several types of drugs in each of the main categories—antipsychotics, mood stabilizers, anxiolytics (targeting anxiety), antidepressants—because when the first drug doesn't help, the next one may, or the one after that, or the one after that. He needs to keep up with new medications when they are introduced. He needs to be conversant with drugs outside the conventional psychiatric categories which are sometimes helpful in treating psychiatric symptoms or medication side effects, for example some hormones, vitamins, and dietary supplements. If his practice is confined mainly to psychotherapy, he at least needs to recognize when medication will be necessary or helpful, and obtain advice from a colleague who is more knowledgeable about pharmacotherapy.

Electroconvulsive Therapy (ECT)

In the first third of the 20th century the bold idea of causing epileptic seizures in mentally ill people as a means of treating their illnesses stemmed from the observation that some people who had both epilepsy and a psychiatric disorder improved temporarily after they had a spontaneous seizure. This, and the mistaken belief that schizophrenia and epilepsy rarely occurred together, led to the deliberate production of seizures in patients—by intravenous injection or inhalation of seizure-producing chemicals or by electric current applied directly to the temples. Only electricity has survived as a safe and effective means of causing seizures in psychiatric treatment. Methods of applying it have been refined and complications from it reduced over the decades since the 1930's, when the Italians Bini and Cerletti developed it. Psychiatrists continue to rely upon it for treating select patients, especially those with severe depression or mania—and some with schizophrenia—who have not improved with medication or whose conditions are so physically and mentally agonizing, or immediately life threatening, that it would be heartless or dangerous to take the slower route of trying medication first.

An electrical current is applied to the head at a charge sufficient to cause brain cells—neurons—to fire and produce a generalized epileptic seizure. The procedure has been refined to the extent that convulsive stiffening and shaking of the body are eliminated by medicines given intravenously just before the seizure. The actions of every one of the neurotransmitters, a class of chemicals responsible for sending impulses from one neuron to another, is affected. If the treatment is successful, then after between six and 12 treatments the patients will improve significantly. Risks of the treatment are no greater than the risks associated with antidepressant medication, not to mention the risk of letting the illness go untreated. To this day, nobody knows why ECT works; but it does, particularly to treat the symptoms of depression and mania.

When ECT began to be used in practice, in the 1940's, it was estimated to relieve the symptoms of depression and mania in over 90% of patients. In those days it was often a first-line treatment, because effective medications for the affective disorders—depression and mania—were not yet in use. By the end of the 20th century the people who received ECT were usually those who had failed treatment with medication. So convulsive therapy is now essentially being offered to people whose illnesses have already demonstrated treatment-resistance. The results of ECT now are thus less gratifying than in the early days of its use.

Be skeptical of anyone who demonizes ECT. Neuropsychological tests have not demonstrated brain damage from this procedure, and it intervenes in life-threatening illnesses. Be skeptical as well of anyone who recommends ECT before using the less-disruptive approaches of medication and psychotherapy, unless the patient's condition is so perilous—from severe agitation, implacable suicidal drive or failure to take food and fluids—that ECT should be the first-line treatment.

COMPASSION

When an applicant to medical school writes her essay on why she has chosen a career as a physician, she will be thought unwise if she doesn't put a desire to help people high on her list of motives. But the members of a school's admissions committee are looking for something more than a warm fuzzy emotion. What has the applicant done to put her altruism into action? Has she spent a semester or summer in the ghettoes of Los Angeles or the shantytowns of Lima, Peru? Has she spent two years as a missionary in the backwoods of the Philippines? Has she sat for hours in a pediatric emergency room, bandaging cuts and comforting crying kids and their frightened or angry parents? What is this applicant made of?

Compassion is kindness in action, empathy with muscle, not simply an emotion. Its opposite is not just mean-spirited feelings, but mean-spirited behavior; and just as tellingly, the opposite of compassion is also a failure to act on behalf of others, whether that failure stems from antipathy or simple laziness.

For the physician in the practice of psychiatry, as for any other physician, compassion means putting the needs of his patient first in his decisions and in the way he acts. It is not so much a matter of emotion as of policy, a deliberate setting of priorities. Altruistic emotions evaporate in the face of a doctor's fatigue, irritation, financial concerns and so forth. He can't count on the continual return of that thrilling love for humanity he first felt as a high school student, volunteering at the local hospital and following the family doctor on her rounds. A stubborn adherence to his decision to act principally on his patients' behalf is his real source of compassion and bulwark against selfishness in the middle of the night when he is faced with a snarling, drunk, mentally ill man, calling him every bad name the doctor ever heard.

The fundamental thing that a physician does is to make decisions concerning her patient. She decides what is wrong and she decides what she is going to do about it, or what she is going to recommend be done about it. These decisions include decisions in the moral sphere, leading to actions which to a greater or lesser extent are driven by compassionate attitudes. Actions on relatively minor issues may reveal the doctor's attitude more convincingly than a thousand words.

The phone rings at 3:00 am. The psychiatrist has been asleep since 12:30. She awakens to the voice of a patient asking her for reassurance about something they had talked about during the office visit two days before. The psychiatrist's first emotion is annoyance—anxiety and its consequent behaviors are often so annoying to others. If the doctor speaks impulsively from that annoyance, she will make the patient feel worse than he already does, undercutting her own fundamental aim to be helpful. If she decides to act from compassion, she must put herself mentally in her patient's place—the place of an anxious man unable to sleep who turns to his doctor for help, so driven by his psychological discomfort that he could not keep his fears to himself until daylight.

As a physician grows in years, he should also grow in wisdom and compassion. This process is aided by his increasing understanding and tolerance of people and their frailties and a sobering awareness of his own fallibility. When the opposite unfortunately occurs, and the doctor becomes increasingly cynical or embittered over the years, the explanation is often to be found in physical or mental afflictions of the doctor himself, or in emotionally shattering events that he has experienced in his professional life.

The practice of psychiatry at times brings the physician face to face with some very angry, irrationally accusatory, cruel, stupid, unfair, slovenly, lazy and selfish people, who are at their absolute worst at the very time when the psychiatrist is called upon to help them. Doing the right thing involves seeking the glory at the center of this person who, whatever the differences between him and the psychiatrist, is in fact more like her than otherwise, by virtue of their shared humanity.

One tragic case haunts me as a failure of compassion in myself, and as a caution about treating members of the same family when they are so divided by bitterness or circumstance that their pathways lie apart.

George, a physician in his 50's came to see me at the insistence of his wife because of his rages that were disrupting the family.

He was successful in his profession, though chronically melancholic and given to excessive drinking. His rages were provoked by trivial things and were always in a domestic setting. On occasion he had struck his wife. A few years into their marriage she had divorced him because of his behavior toward her, only to remarry him soon after in response to his pleadings.

The prescription for his treatment was sobriety, antidepressant mediation, and psycho-therapy. Treatment was successful, though the first two antidepressants we tried had failed, leading to the use of the problematic phenelzine, a monoamine inhibitor. That drug was immediately effective.

Then his 16 year old daughter developed depression, and the couple asked me to treat her too. I agreed, unwisely overlooking the tensions that were building between father and daughter.

All went well until one night when the father ate aged cheese (forbidden for people on MAOI antidepressants). He experienced severe headache from a sudden increase in blood pressure and called me. A visit to an emergency room revealed no stroke or other damage, but I stopped the medication to give him a brief holiday from it because of the hypertensive episode.

Two days later, while he was still without the buffering of his temper afforded by the medication, his daughter defied him by going on a date against his wishes. In the argument that ensued he flew into a rage, wrestled her to the floor, and chopped off most of her long beautiful hair with scissors.

His wife took the daughter and left the house to stay with her sister and called me right away that night. I was furious with him, and had mother and daughter come to my office the next day. The girl was devastated and mortified, and my anger at her father was increased.

If only he, and not also his daughter, had been my patient, I would have called him as soon as I learned of the assault, or at least by the next day, knowing how bitterly guilty and remorseful he always had been after one of his outbursts. I should have called and said something like, "George, you must feel awful. Meet me at the office right now and let's talk about it." But my loyalties were divided. Compassion and clinical judgment were submerged below my anger, and I did nothing to help my patient in this worst crisis of his life. He killed himself the following night with carbon monoxide in his garage.

Respect for her patient and loyalty to him, whether or not he is likable or grateful or possessed of other attractive qualities, undergirds the psychiatrist's compassionate behavior. She works for him, regardless of whether he himself is paying the bill, and his communications must remain in confidence unless to do so will put him or others in danger.

Loyalty is often put to the test, especially when the psychiatrist believes the patient is behaving destructively in his actions toward employer, institution, or another person, or has been engaged in criminal activity. I believe it is in the patient's best interest for the psychiatrist to be questioning, challenging or confrontive in such situations—to be the voice of reality and reason. But I do not believe the psychiatrist should break the patient's confidence, except when it is against the law for a doctor not to do so, as in cases of child abuse, elder abuse and a credible threat against a person.

"Credible" is the key word. Many people make murderous statements in the grips of great emotion. In the great majority of cases the patient is just blowing off steam, but the psychiatrist must question her patient in detail about what he means by his statements. If she thinks there is nothing to it, it is unwise for her to mention it in the patient's record. If she thinks the threat is serious, she must not only mention it in the record but warn the object of the threat as well.

All physicians, psychiatrists included, are in a position to help their patients with matters in their lives beyond the boundaries of the illnesses they are treating them for. Helpful contact with employers, insurance companies, school administrators, social agencies, and so forth—always with the permission of the patients—is entirely within the scope of a psychiatrist's duties, as is limiting the cost of treatment. He should not hesitate to use his influence on his patient's behalf: an excessive amount of detachment is no virtue.

A long-time employee of a large local company was hospitalized for treatment of depression. It was discovered that his symptoms were, to a much greater extent than usual, exquisitely sensitive to changes in his sleep cycle. The patient had tried in vain for years to get his company to regulate his schedule to accommodate this very real biological vulnerability. The patient's psychiatrist phoned the CEO of the company, considered many layers in the hierarchy above the patient, and explained this situation. The CEO acted the same day to effect the schedule change.

Not all such efforts succeed, of course, but the psychiatrist should be faulted if he doesn't at least try in appropriate situations..

A third-year medical student began to behave badly on clinical rounds, arguing loudly with fellow students and house staff. His manner was so obnoxious, that it was viewed as a feature of his personality, not as the symptom of the bipolar disorder that was just beginning. Despite the fact that the young man entered treatment, there was prevalent belief among faculty members that he didn't belong in medical school. The psychiatrist who was treating him then appeared before the governing body of the faculty to plead his case. The student was retained in school, his illness was controlled, and he went on to have a successful career after graduating with his class.

Psychiatrist-Patient Relationship and Its Boundaries

A physician is called upon to think and act on behalf of all his patients with even-handed professionalism. As he grows in his job over the years, he can get better and better at this. He can become progressively more disciplined and more able to find a personal core in his patients to respect and to work with, even when their illnesses or personality features make them unlikable to almost everyone else. In the same way he should be progressively more able to sustain objectivity, and refrain from unprofessional degrees of closeness to those patients whom he finds attractive or with whom he can most easily identify—people who are a lot like him.

The psychiatrist controls the quality boundaries of the doctor-patient relationship. Doctors vary widely in their skills in this respect. Each brings to his medical training his own personal attributes. One student will begin his first contact with patients as bouncy and warm as a puppy, while another will be as cool and aloof as a dignified Siamese cat. Though these two will remain at opposite ends of the warm-cool spectrum during their careers, they should become so tempered by experience, discipline and self-knowledge, that their attitudes and behaviors are at the service of their patients, not a distraction to them.

The key is the amount and the quality of the attention that the doctor is giving to her patient during their encounters. No matter how absorbed in his illness the patient is, he can tell if, and to what degree, the doctor is really paying attention to him. When a psychiatrist doesn't really care about the patient, or is merely indulging her own feelings during the interaction, the patient picks it up.

It is up to the psychiatrist to keep the purpose of the relationship always in mind. Though she may at times get annoyed, even angry, this patient is not her adversary, but someone she is contracted to help if he will let her help him. Though she may be attracted to him, she is not his friend or lover, but his employee. Ideally, patient and psychiatrist like each other and have a friendly relationship. Treatment works best that way. But it is the psychiatrist's responsibility to remember why they are both there, even when the patient forgets it.

Compassionate behavior by the doctor includes striving to understand what the patient needs then helping him get it, while being realistic and kind in the process.

TENACITY

...with its synonyms—persistence, doggedness, perseverance, staying-power—is the essential ingredient for the success of any enterprise, be it winning a ball game or building a cathedral or practicing something more than mediocre psychiatry.

In the majority of psychiatric cases tenacity doesn't come conspicuously into play. Psychiatry is usually not a very difficult specialty to practice. It doesn't bring the over-long hours of family practice and pediatrics and internal medicine, or the physical ardors of general surgery. The psychiatrist is rarely faced with the acute and life-threatening emergencies that are the daily fare of other specialists. The typical clinical psychiatrist works hard, but less hard than most other doctors. The experienced psychiatrist is not greatly challenged by most of her cases.

But then there are the tough cases, where things go badly, or are full of ugly surprises, or drag on into a daunting chronicity. The indispensability of tenacity to the practice of really good psychiatry can be illustrated in its application in three areas: understanding the patients' problems in all their complexity at the beginning of treatment; working with chronically ill patients and those whose illnesses, acute or chronic, resist easy treatment; and cultivating an on-going state of availability to patients, alertness to the possibility of trouble, and avoidance of complacency.

Tenacity in Understanding a Case's Complexity at the Beginning of Treatment

Leon was 17 when he dropped out of school and started to run the streets of his big city and use street drugs more than he had before. During an arrest for peace disturbance he as so conspicuously confused that the police took him to a hospital where he was briefly admitted to the psychiatry division for a few days and given medication until his confusion subsided. Was it drug intoxication only, or did he have a mental illness underlying the symptoms? Nobody found out, because he never followed up with a psychiatrist, and the people the hospital made no effort to contact the family of this wandering boy.

35

Twelve years passed, during which Leon would from time to time show up at the home of various relatives and be a pain in the neck. He was written off as hopeless by his family, and actively ostracized by his brother who was a police officer in the city. He was abused by gangs, even beaten up twice by police, and regarded as an obnoxious loser, probably always on dope. Another arrest when he was 29 led to another brief psychiatric hospitalization, and another course of effective treatment with medication, but no contact with his family and no follow-through on the part of Leon, whose illness deprived him of the capacity to take initiative, whether he was on street drugs or not.

Homeless at age 30, abused in the city's shelters and under the bridges where he sometimes curled up to sleep, one day he showed up at his mother's house. Driven by hallucinated voices telling him that she was a former girlfriend, he choked her and tried to rape her. Once more the police came and took him to a hospital.

The staff at the new hospital did for Leon what had not been done before. They made intensive efforts to contact his family, from whom he had been alienated for years because of his behavior. A more compete history from his reluctant relatives, a negative laboratory screen for street drugs, and a normal MRI of the brain established the diagnosis of schizophrenia. Medication reduced the intensity of the "voices" and eliminated his aggressive urges, but it took a long time and several changes of medication.

Problems remained: where would he go when he was discharged from the hospital? He had no insurance, eliminating the possibility of social services to pay for a group home, community support case management, mental health patient services, or medication. His relatives were afraid of him, and had no understanding of the illness.

These obstacles were overcome by intensive education of his relatives, until his mother agreed to take him in, now that he was no longer delusional; by creative scrounging for samples of medication until his insurance, for which he was entitled because of poverty, became effective; and by free services by his psychiatrist, who had made a special project of his care. After six months he was established in part-time employment in a sheltered workshop, living amicably with his mother, and attending a day program at mental health center.

Leon still had schizophrenia, but he was safe, treated and in the good graces of his family once more. This success stemmed from the psychiatrist's tenacious work of find-

ing out what was really wrong with Leon and convincing his family that there was hope of recovering their lost young man. Without her tenacity, surpassing that of others who had seen him over the previous 13 years, none of these good things would have happened.

Tenacity in Working with Difficult Chronic Cases

Charlotte was probably only in her teens when she began to suffer from periodic spells of depression. By her thirties these had become more painful, and she discovered the short-term relief afforded by marijuana and alcohol. Dependence on them then became a big problem in its own right. Adding to her burden was the fact that her main source of support, her husband, was remote both emotionally and geographically, out of town on business for long stretches.

Nonetheless, she tried to persevere in managing the house and raising their daughter and she began her pursuit of a career in social work by enrolling in graduate school. But despite psychotherapy and medication, she was repeatedly derailed by depression, alcohol, and a growing belief that she was worthless. This was reinforced by her husband's neglect and her own repeated lapses from sobriety. On several occasions over two decades she made serious attempts to kill herself by overdosing on pills, a nearly fatal one after her husband announced he was leaving her.

Things did not begin to turn around until two things happened: her psychiatrist became more aggressive, taking the initiative in tracking her down if she missed an appointment, pushing her to maintain her substance-abuse recovery program, and adjusting her complex medication regimen more promptly—as soon as a combination of drugs had demonstrated itself to be insufficiently effective; and her 18 year old daughter became pregnant by a fleeting acquaintance and elected to keep the baby, conferring on Charlotte a new indispensability.

Maintenance of a satisfactory level of wellness by Charlotte was now underway.

Tenacity in Maintaining Availability

Two of my own cases illustrate the importance of a psychiatrist's availability, and the tragic consequences that can follow when his availability is insufficient.

Cheryl was 11 when she developed anorexia nervosa, a self-starvation which lasted for a year then went away on its own. In her mid-teens she began to have episodes of depression and a recurrence of eating disorder—obsessions with her weight with food-binging followed by purging by vomiting. She became my patient when she was 16. Now she is 36.

Finding an effective combination of medication and supportive psychotherapy for this chronic illness was the easy part. The keys to her maintenance of a endurable life have been her stubborn persistence in pursuing the goal of wellness, and my availability to her, in person, by phone and e-mail, wherever she happened to be and at all hours. During these 20 years she has had depressions, suicide attempts, bulimic episodes, bad boyfriends, diet pill abuse, several moves to states far away, job changes, a successful search for her birth-mother, solidifying relations with her adoptive parents, a stable marriage, miscarriages, and now finally a pregnancy carried to term. Through all this she has not given up. Cheryl will never be free of susceptibility to depression and bulimia nervosa, but she has the tools to manage these disorders and a support system of many people she can count on to be there for her.

Every psychiatrist has tales like that to tell. They make it all worth it.

Then there was Robert.

Robert was 35 when he first came to be treated for anxiety in the 1980's. He was a tall, single, athletic young man, a golf pro at a local country club. He was something of a hypochondriac, fretting about his health in general, and recurrently obsessed with a fear of AIDS, which had just begun to receive widespread publicity. After each sexual encounter with his girlfriend he had begun to fret and to question her fidelity. He was easily reassured, it seemed to me at the time, and a medication for anxiety helped. I underestimated the degree to which he could distort realty and his need for greater availability than I was providing.

His health worries were not without foundation, because somewhere along he line had acquired hepatitis-C. An infectious disease specialist began treatment with interferon, an anti-viral drug that can cause depression. I went blithely on, seeing him every few months, though he needed to be seen with much greater frequency, and I needed to emphasize more emphatically that I was available to him between appointments.

Then one day I read his obituary in the morning paper. I phoned his mother who told me that he had become very depressed, convinced that he had AIDS and would die a horrible death, and had shot himself.

I blame myself. He could have been saved.

The psychiatrist's tenacity can be limited, and eroded by fatigue, shortage of time, and pessimism about a case. We can also find many excuses for giving up or settling for too little, especially when our patients' own perseverance and capacity for optimism are undermined by their illnesses or by sad circumstances in their lives. Though we are never perfect when it comes to tenacity, we are not absolved from doggedly continuing to pursue our, and our patients', vision of wellness and wholeness, insofar as they may be attainable. I believe that a psychiatrist's ability to be tenacious in her work exceeds her capacity to be knowledgeable and compassionate, derived as it is from the same primitive drive that is essential for survival. Finally, it is incumbent on her to realize that the patient's tenacity is even more essential to success than the psychiatrist's tenacity, and that she, along with other supporting people, must lead the way in that respect. If doctors aren't tenacious, they can't expect their patients to be.

CONCLUSION

This short book discusses what I believe are the essential elements of the practice of good psychiatry—or of good medicine in general, for that matter: knowledge, compassion, and tenacity. I believe that these principles are enduring, and that they were as relevant for healers thousands of years ago as they are for physicians today.

The idea is hardly original. Good doctors have always figured it out for themselves, and tried their best to live up to these and other principles of excellent practice. The present book gives examples of how they can be applied to the treatment of people who suffer from psychiatric disorders. I wanted to bring this to the attention of patients and their families, to further their understanding of what to expect their physicians to strive for. No psychiatrist practices these principles perfectly, of course, but the best ones try hardest.

Richard W. Hudgens, M.D.
Professor of Psychiatry
Washington University School of Medicine
St. Louis, Missouri

0-595-33542-X

www.ingramcontent.com/pod-product-compliance
Lightning Source LLC
Chambersburg PA
CBHW021043180526
45163CB00005B/2263